BEI GRIN MACHT SICH IHR WISSEN BEZAHLT

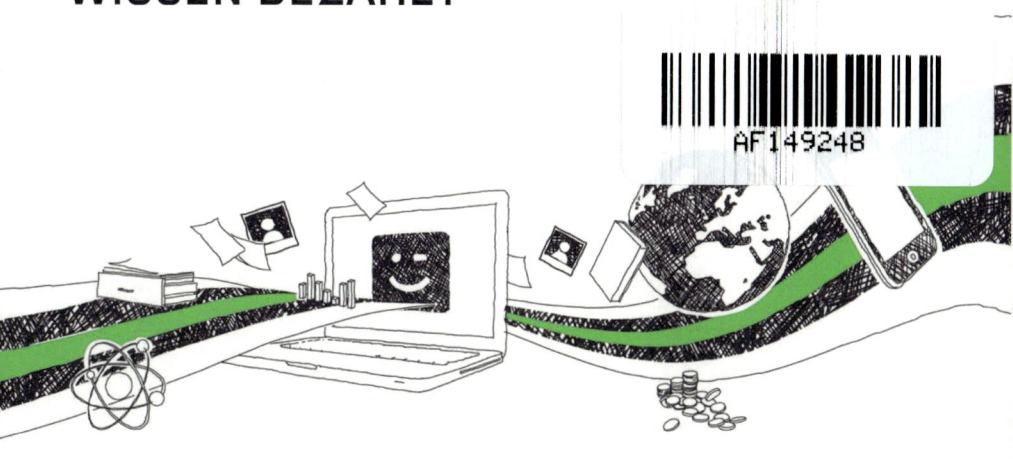

- Wir veröffentlichen Ihre Hausarbeit, Bachelor- und Masterarbeit

- Ihr eigenes eBook und Buch - weltweit in allen wichtigen Shops

- Verdienen Sie an jedem Verkauf

Jetzt bei www.GRIN.com hochladen und kostenlos publizieren

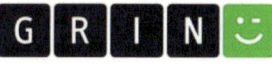

Yun Feng, Yang Li, Wei Wang

Reduced wavefront aberration influence the visual function after the senile cataract surgery with an aspherical intraocular lens

GRIN Verlag

Bibliografische Information der Deutschen Nationalbibliothek:

Die Deutsche Bibliothek verzeichnet diese Publikation in der Deutschen National-
bibliografie; detaillierte bibliografische Daten sind im Internet über http://dnb.d-
nb.de/ abrufbar.

Impressum:

Copyright © 2013 GRIN Verlag GmbH
Druck und Bindung: Books on Demand GmbH, Norderstedt Germany
ISBN: 978-3-656-42218-1

Dieses Buch bei GRIN:

http://www.grin.com/de/e-book/213709/reduced-wavefront-aberration-influence-
the-visual-function-after-the-senile

GRIN - Your knowledge has value

Der GRIN Verlag publiziert seit 1998 wissenschaftliche Arbeiten von Studenten, Hochschullehrern und anderen Akademikern als eBook und gedrucktes Buch. Die Verlagswebsite www.grin.com ist die ideale Plattform zur Veröffentlichung von Hausarbeiten, Abschlussarbeiten, wissenschaftlichen Aufsätzen, Dissertationen und Fachbüchern.

Besuchen Sie uns im Internet:

http://www.grin.com/

http://www.facebook.com/grincom

http://www.twitter.com/grin_com

REDUCED WAVEFRONT ABERRATION INFLUENCE THE VISUAL FUNCTION AFTER THE SENILE CATARACT SURGERY WITH AN ASPHERICAL INTRAOCULAR LENS

Yun Feng, Yang Li, Wei Wang

The ophthalmology department of the 3rd teaching hospital of Peking University, Peking University Eye Center, Beijing 100083

Purpose: To evaluate whether the aspherical intraocular lens (IOL) with a modified aspherical anterior surface provides better quality of vision than the conventional spherical IOL for the senile cataract patients after phacoemusification and IOL implantation.

Methods: Consecutively 115 eyes were selected from 72 senile cataract patients who received phacoemulsification and IOL implantation in Peking University Eye Center, age range from 49 to 84(63.9 ± 9.9 years old).Each was randomly assigned to receive TecnisZ9001 IOL or CeeOnEdge 911 and or Sensar AR40e (both made by AMO). In the time frame from one day before operation, one week, one month, three months and six months after operation, the eyes underwent several checkups by the same personnel. checkups included visual acuity, optometry, contrast sensitivity test and wavefront aberration (WA) examination. The parameters included best corrective visual acuity, the values of contrast sensitivity, Z_4^0 Zernike coefficient, root mean square of the 4th order (RMS4) and higher-order root mean square (RMSh). Visual functional questionnaires were finished and the scores were saved. Then statistical analysis needs to be done.

Results: Spherical wavefront aberration has positive correlation with the age ($r=0.582$, P value<0.05). There are no significant difference of BCVA between each two of the three groups before or after the operation (P value>0.05). The patients with Tecnis IOL get lower Z40 Zernike coefficient, RMS4 and the RMSh than these items in the CeeOn 911 group and Sensar AR40e group(P value<0.05), and higher contrast sensitivity at the 5 level of spatial frequency. Furthermore, the visual function scores are higher than the other two spherical IOL group (P value<0.05).

Conclusion: The older of the patient, the higher spherical wavefront of the eye would be. Different from the conventional spherical IOL, a kind of aspherical IOL can provide better quality of vision by reducing the spherical wavefront after cataract surgery.

Key Words: Intraocular lens, aberration, cataract, visual function

Corresponding author: Wei Wang,

The human eyes are not ideal optical devices. In theory, size and space differences of photoreceptor cells make it possible for the retinal resolution to reach $3.0^{[1,2]}$. Due to the existence of wavefront aberration which limits the visual quality, BCVA can only reach 2.0 or lower. Despite conventional refractive surgeries do make corrections with satisfying postoperative vision, many patients complain about the syndrome and side-effects associated with the surgery, such as dizzying, selaphobia, lowered contrast sensitivity, blurred vision in dark environment etc. Research has found that the postoperative vision weakening is related to the increase of higher-order aberration. Study of wavefront aberration of the human eyes, especially higher-order aberrations, is something new that was developed in recent years. Its clinical application mainly reflects in refractive surgeries that are driven by wavefront aberration. In clinical terms, the aberrations are occasioned by cornea and lens. Along with aging, the aberration also grows. If spherical IOLs are implanted in a cataract surgery, positive aberration may still occur,

which will not eliminate corneal aberration. The emerging intraocular lens, however, results in negative spherical aberration. With special treatments to the anterior/posterior chambers of the corneal lens, corneal refractivity will be reduced and therefore it compensates the positive corneal aberration.

Our research focuses on comparing differences between spherical and aspherical IOL to patients' visual function after senile cataract surgery, especially emphasizing on the study of postoperative spherical aberrations. Results from objective and subjective observations are carefully studied. Other parameters, including the best corrective visual acuity, the values of contrast sensitivity and questionnaires collecting results of patients' vision after surgery, are all applied in the analysis of our research.

1. Objects & Methodology
1.1 Objects of Study

From February to December 2005, 72 patients diagnosed cataract by and treated in the Peking University Eye Center with a total of 115 eyes were the major objects of the study. Among them, 43 patients received cataract surgeries on both eyes. For statistics and figures please refer to Table1. As our research requires a keen cooperation from the patients in postoperative checkups on parameters such as the values of contrast sensitivity, the result of subjective aberration checkups, the patients' occupation, education level, therefore, matters. Such results from follow-up checkups as a matter of fact play a key role in weighting our study. After analyzing the characteristics and traits of the clan of our patients, with our Eye Center's geographic location and surrounding habitant composition in mind, we narrowed down our research participates to those who mostly were retiree teachers and governmental officers as this clan of patients normally enjoy a relatively higher education level. We also invited retirees who would like to cooperate with us on after-surgery follow-ups. Due to limited resources of our Eye Center, however, we cannot guarantee a completely random-chosen mechanism in terms of pinning down each patient. We tried our best to assure the continuity of our cases. Detailed screening criterion please refers to in the following **Participants chosen criterion** (1.4) and the principle that same IOL should be used on both eyes on a single patient applies throughout our research.

	Person	Eyes	Age± standard deviation	Age (lower limit)	Age (upper limit)	Gaussian distribution
Total	72	115	63.9±9.9	49	84	Yes
TecnisZ9001	37	55	65.2±10.4	50	84	Yes
CeeOn911	19	28	61.4±9.4	49	83	Yes
Sensar	16	32	64.0±9.1	51	76	Yes

Table1. Case scenario TecnisZ9001，CeeOn911and Sensar materials are used in three groups of patients respectively with participants' age range between 49-84 years-old, average 63.9 years-old, in line with the mathematical approach as normal distribution.

1.2 Research Material
1.2.1 Intraocular lens
- TecnisZ9001, AMO（Advanced Medical Optics）(US firm)
- CeeOn Edge911, AMO (US firm)
- Sensar AR40e, AMO (US firm)

1.2.2 Devices

- Standard logarithmic vision chart and Jaeger vision chart
- FACT test card for the measuring of contrast sensitivity
- Noncontact tonometer: Canon, Tonometer TX-10
- Cornea curvimeter: Nikon, Speedy-K
- counts of corneal endothelium, Iconan, Nonconrobo Pachy
- A-type ultrasonic device: Alcon, The Ultrascan Imaging System
- corneal keratometer, Zeiss, WaveLight, Allegro Topolyzer
- Subjective wave-front aberrometer: WFA1000 from Suzhou Liangjing Medical Equipment Co., ltd
- Objective wavefront aberrometer: Zeiss, WaveLight, Allegretto Wave Analyzer
- Sovereign phacoemulsification instrument: AMO Co., ltd USA

1.3 Methodology

1.3.1 Checkups before-surgery include:

☐ Uncorrected far/near visual acuity

☐ Standard optometry, best corrective and uncorrective visual acuity

☐ Tonometer: 3 consecutive measures should be taken using Tonometer TX-10 noncontact tonometer, high and low margins are balanced within 3mm range, the mean should be taken

☐ Rountain slit lamp and fundus examination;

☐ Corneal diopter measures: Speedy-K diopter measuring device should be used with the parameter of 12mm, high and low margins are indicated as K1 and K2 respectively; the high point and low point are used in the calculation of IOL modeling;

☐ Counts of corneal endothelium cells: Nonconrobo Pachy non-contact device should be used: cell density on the medium, on point-3 and point-9 should be recorded together with the percentage of hexagonal cell;

☐ Axial length measuring: 10MHz A-type device should be used, result will be used in determining IOL;

☐ Corneal topology test: Allegro Topolyzer should be used to exam lesions other than ailments on the corneal curvature and keratoconus etc.

☐ Subjective aberration test: WFA1000 Subjective aberration measuring device should be used, the patient should conduct such tests on themselves. Method will be taught to the patients and three times of tests should be observed for the best result;

☐ Objective wavefront aberration test: Allegretto Wave Analyzer objective aberration testing device should be used; Mydriatic eye drop should be used on the sick eye(s) 10min/doses ×3～5 doses; 10 minutes after the last dose when the diameter of the pupil is larger than 6.0mm, an objective aberration test should be conducted. All such tests should be conducted by the same person with at least 4 times of each tests done so on the same eye so as to screen out one best result that satisfies the following criterions: 1) lowest dispersion value between the lower-order aberration (myopic astigmatism) and the optometry result; 2) best match of the high-order aberration graph and the root mean square; 3) best focus of the original photo; 4) lest dislocation from the center. The focal point of our research is the result of objective wavefront aberration. Thanks to the software studying condition of the eye, we can observe various level of aberrations occurred in different miotic conditions (with different pupil diameters)

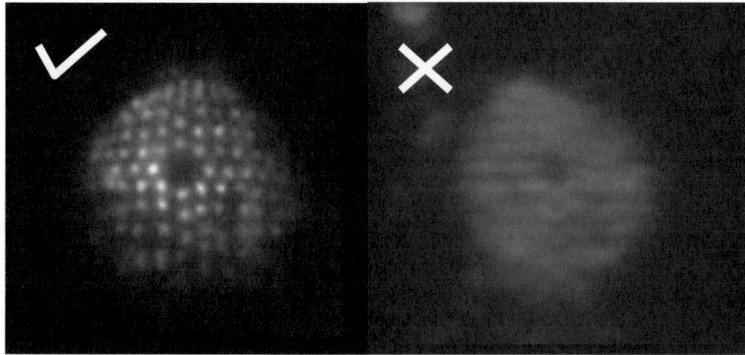

Graph1. Analysis on typical wavefronts

☐ FACT test on contrast sensitivity: exam the intensity of light on a fixed location, record the contrast sensitivity on patients in a natural light environment with the tests conducted by the same person, five clusters of parameters (1.5—18c/deg) are recorded (Graph 2)

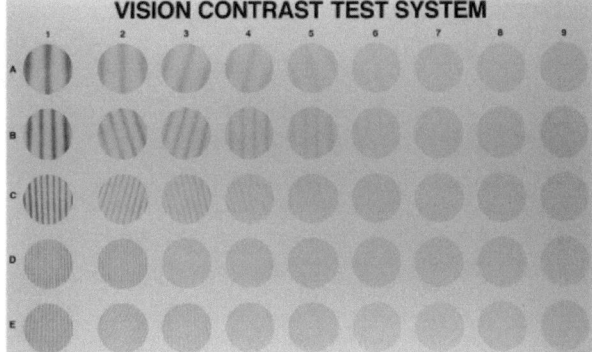

Graph2. FACT Chart comparison on the contrast sensitivity

☐ Subjective visual psychological scaling: A postoperative visual function measuring table modified from VF —14 should be used (Table3). Worldwide, VF—14 is the most widely used measurement on visual function in the subjective measuring approach[3,4.] Research participants are required to give scores to the easiness of 14 items that they encounter everyday. Easiness of completing such daily conducts is divided into five degrees with certain points assigned: no difficulty in completing the whole daily conduct = 100 points; almost no difficulty = 75 points; difficult to complete = 50 points, with material difficulty = 25 points; impossible to achieve such tasks = 0 points; the visual function is measured by the final points collected on each individual. Because of cultural differences, however, the original version of such tests is not in line with the social practice in China and therefore, based on the standard VF-14, we made some changes on the first, second and twelfth items of the questionnaire and came up with a new table as the measurement of after-surgery visual function on each patient. The higher total points a patient may collect means his/her after-surgery visual function is finer.[5]

Table3. VF−14 and after-surgery visual function level

VF−14		Postoperative visual function
1.	Drive in daytime	Ride a bike in daytime
2.	Drive in nighttime	Ride a bike in the evening
3.		read labels, prescriptions written on the packages of food and drugs
4.		reading
5.	Read headlines on a newspaper or texts in larger font, keys on a telephone	
6.		Identify people approaching
7.		identify stairs
8.		Identify traffic signs, read trademarks on a
supermarket/drugstore		
9.		sewing, knitting, woodcraft and/or other handcrafting tasks
10.		Looking for particular items
11.		Play poker games and/or mah-jong
12.	Play golf, tennis	Fly a kit, play gateball
13.		cooking
14.		watch TV

1.3.2 Methodology of Surgery

☐ Preparation: oflaxin eye drop Qid should be used 3 days before the operation, upon surgery, no need to remove eyelashes before surgery, clearance of lacrimal passage needs to be confirmed; clean the conjunctival sac with water; mydriatic eye drop Q15′×4 times; anesthetic extender should be made by a mix of same volume 2% lidocanine and 0.75% bubicanine, a 3−3.5ml dose should be injected.

☐ Procedure: standard sanitization before surgery, protective film should be used; transparent corneal incision were made at 11 o'clock and 2 o'clock, standard procedure for phacoemulcification。

☐ Postoperative treatment: orally antibiotics and topical steroids were used(Debrax,Alcon, Qid) combined preparation。

1.3.3 Postoperative checkups and follow-ups

Postoperative checkups cover 6 months after surgery and are conduced on the first week, first month, third month and sixth month respectively. Each checkup includes measuring of uncorrected vision, best corrective visual acuity and intraocular pressure; using slit lamp to exam parameters such as the healing degree of the surgical incisions, ailments in the anterior chamber, the depth of the anterior chamber, size of the pupil; the location of intraocular lens, the completeness of the posterior chamber; direct and indirect ophthalmoscope and funduscopy tests should be conducted in order to exam the condition of vitreous, the chorioretian condition and to see if macular edema may occur. We pay more attention on the anterior chamber depth since it is related to the aberration. Corneal topology and subjective/objective aberration checkups should be made on the first month, the third month and the sixth month after the surgery respectively. The questionnaire program should be kicked off after 3 months of surgery so as to collect relevant information on the patients' contrast sensitivity and his/her visual psychological results.

1.4 Participants chosen criterion:

☐ Age between 45-85 years-old;

☐ In sound mental and physical condition, cooperative with follow-up checkups

☐ With sound physical condition, no severe visceral disorders/failures; physical condition allows a cataract surgery and no recent drug usage history that may have an effect on the vision, no recent take of drugs such as Digitalis etc;

5

- No any other ophthalmic disorders than senile cataract;
- Pre-surgery or after-surgery mydriatic level reaches or higher than 6mm;
- Patient remains sound condition during the surgery; stable anterior chamber, no hemorrhage; diameter of curvilinear capsulorhexis is circa 4.5-6mm; complete posterior chamber; intraocular lens implanted into the chamber with correct positions;
- No injury during the postoperative checkup, with stable intraocular pressure; clear cornea; cycloidal pupil; intraocular lens in right position; vitreous, retina with no obvious lesions
- No PCO occurs after 6 months after surgery

1.5 Methodology of Statistics

- A linear correlation is found between the age of patient and his/her wavefront aberration visual psychological scaling;
- Compare the pre-surgery visual psychological scalings (VPS) from aspherical IOLs; compare differences between subjective and objective spherical aberrations; conduct t-test on the two groups of individual samplings;
- Compare each intraocular lens pre-surgery and after-surgery; compare VPS results take in three month after surgery; conduct in-pair t-test;
- Compare subjective/objective spherical aberration differences of each intraocular lens, analyze results collected in the time slot as pre-surgery, 1 month after, 3 month after and 6 month after; conduct in-pair t-test;
- Compare VPS collected after 3 months after surgery on each intraocular lens (spherical and aspherical) and conduct two group of t-test;
- Compare aberration differences collected on 1 month, 3 months, 6 months after surgery (both spherical and aspherical) on different intraocular lens and conduct two group of individual sampling t-test;
- Compare contrast sensitivity differences observed 3-month before/after surgery on different IOLs (both spherical and aspherical); analyze the comparison by means of SPSS 11.5;

2. Result

2.1 Analysis on the correlation of age and pre-surgery testing results

75 patients, 115 eyes, age range between 49~84 with average age 63.9±9.9 years-old are studied. An obvious linear correlation is observed between age and VPS index （607.2±267.8）. The study of pre-surgery objective aberration indicates that age and wavefront aberration Z_4^0 （0.388±0.109μm）and RMS4 （0.591±0.200）are linear correlated. At the meantime, age and overall aberration RMSh （1.313±0.670）are significantly correlated（P value lower than 0.005）（Graph 3-6）。

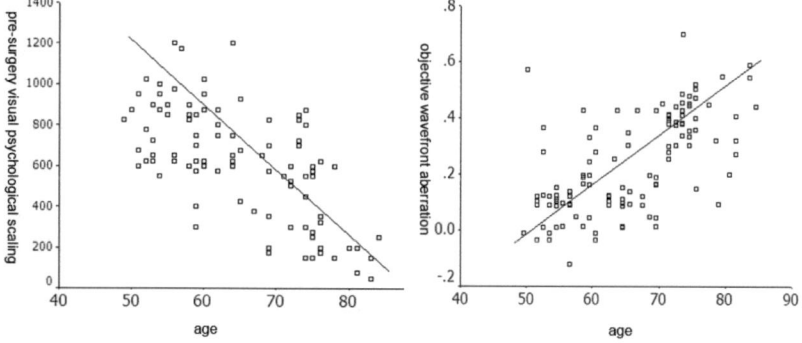

Figure 3. Left, Correlation of age (x-axis) and pre-surgery visual psychological scaling (y-axis), r=−0.668, P=0.000<0.05

Figure 4 Right, Correlation of age (x-axis) and pre-surgery objective wavefront aberration (y-axis) Z40, r=0.582, P=0.006 <0.05

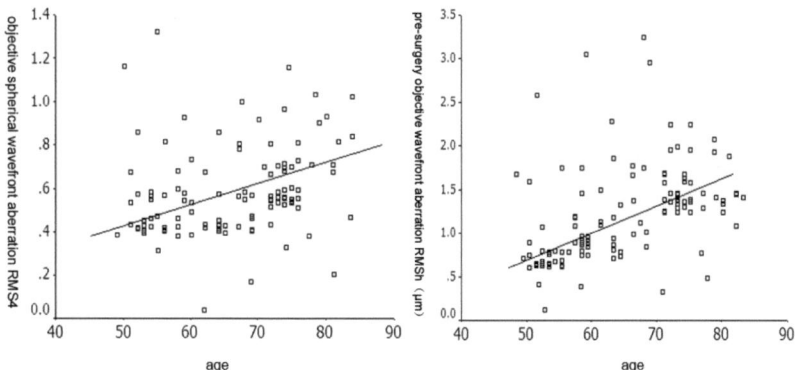

Figure 5 Left, Correlation of age (x-axis) and pre-surgery objective spherical wavefront aberration RMS4 (y-axis), r=0.472, P=0.01<0.05

Figure 6 Right, Correlation of age (x-axis) and pre-surgery objective wavefront aberration RMSh (μm) (y-axis), r=0.534, P=0.000<0.003

2.2 Pre-surgery VPS and comparison of subjective objective aberrations

Comparisons are made of pre/post surgery group Tecnis and Group 911; as well as Group Tecnisand and Group Sensar; P_{T-9} and P_{T-S} represent the individual P value as shown in Table 4. No statistical differences observed.

Table 4. Pre-surgery parameters and subjective/objective aberration

Item	Tecnis	911	P_{T-9}	Sensar	P_{T-S}
Visual psychological scaling	637.7±261.6	571.4±322.3	0.174	585.9±225.0	0.068
Objective Z_4^0 (μm)	0.418±0.112	0.556±0.317	0.093	0.473±0.233	0.118
Objective RMS4 (μm)	0.622±0.230	0.654±0.293	0.530	0.565±0.200	0.452
Objective RMSh (μm)	1.171±0.855	1.228±0.990	0.672	1.235±0.843	0.372
Subjective Z_4^0 (μm)	0.575±0.291	0.525±0.337	0.823	0.625±0.390	0.158
Subjective RMS4 (μm)	0.804±0.331	0.877±0.305	0.099	0.769±0.385	0.682
Subjective RMSh (μm)	1.427±0.670	1.561±0.751	0.062	1.625±0.811	0.295

2.3 VPS comparison of each group 3-month before/after surgery

As Table5 shows, cataract surgery can significantly improve the visual function of the eye(s) of the patient

7

Table5. VPS scores before/after surgery

Group	Pre-surgery score	3-month after surgery score	P
Tecnis	637.7±261.6	1169±211.2	0.045
911	571.4±322.3	1094±293.8	0.000
Sensar	585.9±225.0	1031±189.5	0.006

2.4 Subjective/objective aberrations of each group collected on the first month, 3 months, or 6 months after surgery

2.4.1 All parameters in group Tecnis indicate the existing of material differences in statistical terms; shown as Table5

Table 5. Subjective/Objective aberrations before surgery of Group Tecnis

	Objective aberration（μm）			Subjective aberration（μm）		
	Z_4^0	RMS4	RMSh	Z_4^0	RMS4	RMSh
pre-surgery	0.418±0.112	0.622±0.230	1.171±0.855	0.575±0.291	0.804±0.331	1.427±0.670
1-month after	0.0872±0.173	0.341±0.305	0.642±0.600	0.410±0.309	0.625±0.417	0.986±0.735
P value	0.001	0.005	0.02	0.009	0.04	0.01
Material difference	V	V	V	V	V	V
3 months after	0.111±0.098	0.381±0.296	0.589±0.475	0.363±0.391	0.714±0.606	1.001±0.774
P value	0.006	0.01	0.02	0.02	0.04	0.02
Material difference	V	V	V	V	V	V
6 months after	0.099±0.103	0.318±0.186	0.609±0.345	0.300±0.325	0.619±0.633	0.845±1.062
P value	0.009	0.01	0.03	0.04	0.04	0.03
Material difference	V	V	V	V	V	V

V indicates that statistical difference may apply

2.4.2　911 Key parameters of objective and subjective aberrations comparison before and after surgery, shown as Table 6.

Table 6. Group 911 Objective and subjective aberrations before and after surgery

	Objective aberration（μm）			Subjective aberration（μm）		
	Z_4^0	RMS4	RMSh	Z_4^0	RMS4	RMSh
pre-surgery	0.556±0.317	0.654±0.293	1.228±0.990	0.525±0.337	0.877±0.305	1.561±0.751
1-month after	0.601±0.875	1.141±0.699	1.503±0.970	0.239±0.288	0.922±0.667	1.186±0.867
P value	0.12	0.374	0.09	0.04	0.304	0.08
Material difference	X	X	X	V	X	X
3 months after	0.443±0.248	0.859±0.660	1.222±1.090	0.409±0.518	0.741±0.660	1.335±0.808
P value	0.24	0.152	0.317	0.601	0.100	0.476
Material difference	X	X	X	X	X	X
6 months after	0.509±0.472	0.718±0.504	1.038±0.811	0.611±0.427	0.669±0.450	1.299±1.126
P value	0.342	0.06	0.470	0.223	0.102	0.085
Material difference	X	X	X	X	X	X

V indicates that statistical difference may apply; X indicates no statistical difference applies;

One month after surgery subjective aberration Z_4^0 decreased compared with that tested pre-surgery; no significant statistical differences between the figure collected on the third month and on the sixth month after surgery; other items are with no statistical significance.

2.4.3 No statistical differences of objective/subjective aberrations before or after surgery in Group Sensar, shown as Table 7

Table 7. Objective/subjective aberration observed in Group Sensar before/after surgery

	Objective aberration (μm)			Subjective aberration (μm)		
	Z_4^0	RMS4	RMSh	Z_4^0	RMS4	RMSh
pre-surgery	0.473±0.233	0.565±0.200	1.235±0.843	0.625±0.390	0.769±0.385	1.625±0.811
1 months after	0.582±0.610	0.616±0.453	1.441±1.107	0.710±0.355	0.801±0.714	1.689±1.375
P value	0.08	0.11	0.31	0.50	0.09	0.51
Material difference	X	X	X	X	X	X
3 months after	0.610±0.587	0.499±0.5276	1.110±1.210	0.633±0.412	0.772±0.590	1.446±0.9804
P value	0.241	0.19	0.615	0.31	0.10	0.24
Material difference	X	X	X	X	X	X
6 months after	0.557±0.632	0.618±0.628	1.219±0.905	0.700±0.355	0.719±0.633	1.754±1.162
P value	0.22	0.09	0.16	0.12	0.46	0.38
Material difference	X	X	X	X	X	X

X indicates no statistical difference is observed

2.5 VPS scores comparison on different intraocular lens, collected on 3 months after surgery
comparison of Group Tecnis and Group 911; Group Tecnis and Group Sensar on data collected 3 months after surgery; t-test is made with no statistical differences observed;

Table8. 3 months after surgery VPS scores on different intraocular lens

Tecnis	911	P_{T-9}	Sensar	P_{T-S}
1169±211.2	1094±293.8	0.01	1031±189.5	0.008

2.6 Best corrective visual acuities collected on each group on 1-month, 3-month and 6-month before/after surgery
No statistical differences are observed in Group Tecnis and Group 911, no statistical differences are observed in Group Tecnis and Group Sensar.

2.7 Subjective/objective aberration comparison of different intraocular lens collected on 1-month, 3-month and 6-month after surgery

2.7.1 Subjective/Objective aberration collected on 1-month after surgery
Illustrated as Table 9, statistical differences are seen in Group Tecnis and Group 911 as well as Group Tecnis and Group Sensar

Table 9. Each group subjective objective aberrations on 1-month after surgery

	Objective aberration （μm）			Subjective aberration （μm）		
	Z_4^0	RMS4	RMSh	Z_4^0	RMS4	RMSh
Tecnis	0.0872±0.173	0.341±0.305	0.642±0.600	0.410±0.309	0.625±0.417	0.986±0.735
911	0.601±0.875	1.141±0.699	1.503±0.970	0.239±0.288	0.922±0.667	1.186±0.867
P_{T-9}	0.005	0.010	0.001	0.046	0.039	0.001
Sensar	0.582±0.610	0.616±0.453	1.441±1.107	0.710±0.355	0.801±0.714	1.689±1.375
P_{T-S}	0.012	0.024	0.030	0.005	0.040	0.009

2.7.2   Comparison of subjective/objective aberrations at 3-month after surgery

As Table 10 illustrated, results from Group Tecnis and Group 911, results from Group Tecnis and Group Sensar indicate the existing of statistical differences; in the results collected after 3 months after surgery, Z_4^0 of Group Tecnis and that of Group 911 and RMS4 are no statistical differences; RMS4 from Group Tecnis and Group Sensar are with no statistical differences.

Table 10.   Subjective/Objective aberrations after 3 months of surgery

	Objective aberration （μm）			Subjective aberration （μm）		
	Z_4^0	RMS4	RMSh	Z_4^0	RMS4	RMSh
Tecnis	0.111±0.098	0.381±0.296	0.589±0.475	0.363±0.391	0.714±0.606	1.001±0.774
911	0.443±0.248	0.859±0.660	1.222±1.090	0.409±0.518	0.741±0.660	1.335±0.808
P_{T-9}	0.020	0.018	0.006	0.158	0. 893	0.022
Sensar	0.610±0.587	0.499±0.5276	1.110±1.210	0.633±0.412	0.772±0.590	1.446±0.9804
P_{T-S}	0.008	0.044	0.003	0.035	0.059	0.040

2.7.3   Comparison of subjective objective aberration collected 6 months after surgery

Table 11.   Subjective and objective aberrations after 6 months of surgery

	Objective aberration （μm）			Subjective aberration （μm）		
	Z_4^0	RMS4	RMSh	Z_4^0	RMS4	RMSh
Tecnis	0.099±0.103	0.318±0.186	0.609±0.345	0.300±0.325	0.619±0.633	0.845±1.062
911	0.509±0.472	0.718±0.504	1.038±0.811	0.611±0.427	0.669±0.450	1.299±1.126
P_{T-9}	0.001	0.028	0.016	0.048	0. 636	0.142
Sensar	0.557±0.632	0.618±0.628	1.219±0.905	0.700±0.355	0.719±0.633	1.754±1.162
P_{T-S}	0.000	0.024	0.029	0.035	0.059	0.080

As illustrated by Table11, aberrations observed from Group Tecnis and Group911, as well as results from Group Tecnis and Group Sensar are with statistical differences; RMS4 and RMSh observed 6 months after surgery in Group Tecnis and Group 911 are with no statistical differences; RMS4 and RMSh in Group Tecnis and those of Group Sensar are also with no statistical differences.

2.8   Contrast sensitivity comparisons on intraocular lens made one month, three months and six months before/after surgery, shown as Graph 7

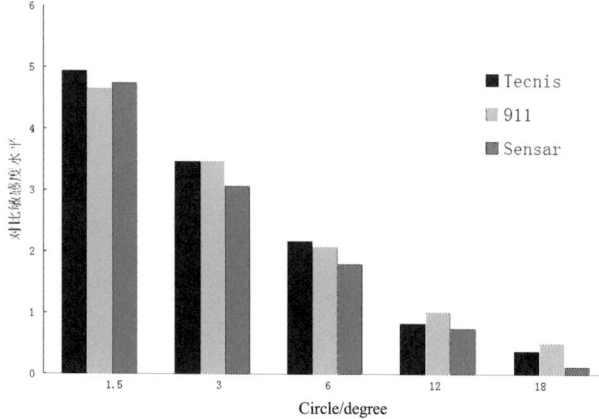

Graph7. Contrast sensitivity comparisons on three groups of intraocular lens

2.8.2   Sensitivity comparisons made 3 months after surgery, shown as Graph 8:

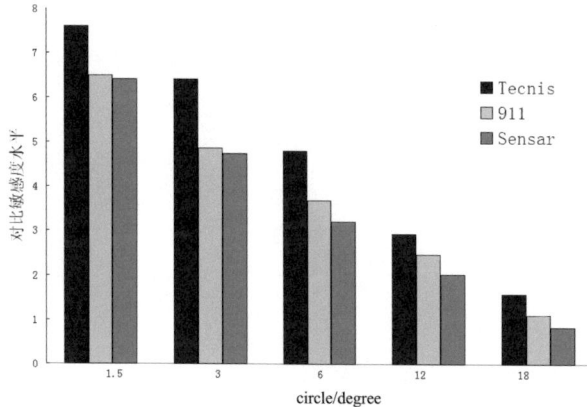

Graph 8. Comparison of contrast sensitivity on three clans of intraocular lens after 3 months of surgery

3. Discussion

Difference is observed by comparing the wavefronts generated by the light matrix with that of an ideal wavefront. Brown and Wolf named this difference as the wavefront aberration. Wavefront aberration may vary significantly [6]. By looking into the aberration or aberration combinations that the human eye system is possible to support, measuring by wavelength, we can further investigate changes of wavefront aberrations and the image detected by the eye when such changes occur [7]. Currently various measurements have been introduced to not only measure but simulate or recreate typical aberrations such as spherical aberrations, defocus aberrations, astigmatism, coma aberrations etc. With these new methods, some irregular aberrations can also be measured [8,9]. In this way, it makes possible to analyze all sorts of aberrations in an ophthalmic fashion and therefore to better assess the visual

functional quality. For example, in the Gull-strand model, aberration and a point-spread-function can be tracked back by a light path, which shows that the best resolution for images received by retina would happen when the diameter of the pupil reaches 2~3mm. After adjustments are made on the aberration, for pupil with the diameter circa 8mm[10] We may conclude that by measuring and correcting the wavefront aberration accurately, not only the vision may reach 20/10 or higher, we can better conduct ourselves in a corneal refractive surgery with precision on the cutting area or to better adjust the aberration on the patient's eyes after surgery. That's also the reason that we pay close attention to experiments on wavefront aberration and its subsequent clinical values.

Age caused cataracts are the main contributor to the downgrade of visual function. Cataract surgery, therefore, provides a good opportunity for senior patients to improve their vision. Thanks to a higher level of comfort living offered by the modern society, patients demand has also surged from "able to see" to "see it crystal clear". Thanks to the renovation in material and technology in IOL, cataract surgery has also been updated to a level that provides a better visual function for patients. This technology, i.e. improving wavefront aberration by means of IOL so as to uplift visual quality, becomes the center of attention. Our study – by comparing aberrations after surgeries where different types of IOL are used – links wavefront aberration with after-surgery visual quality. We further press on the importance of wavefront aberration in terms of cataract surgery and the future development of IOL technology.

3.1 Measurement of wavefront aberrations
Information captured by subjective wavefront aberration instrument is actually generated by visual neurons located on the fundus retina, which is relatively reliable. Such test, however, falls into the psychological physics category which means that the credibility very much relies on the patients' cooperation and their level of comprehension. On the other hand, wavefront aberration, as a subject matter, is also in a constant changing manner[11] Changes of the pupil, strengthening or weakening of adjustment may all interfere the test results. So far no universal standard on the accuracy of the test results is available yet. Our research requires that the refractive degree detected by the WA device should be in line with subjective optometry so as to correct high-order aberration based on a refractive fix. In addition, it also requires that the patient's pupil diameter should be no longer than 5mm, optical area of surgery 6mm. This is to offset the effect of pupil to the result of our after-surgery checkup. We found that the reliability of test results, the level of cooperation may differ significantly even among patients who are in exact same age range; each subjective WA result may also significantly differ from one another.

Allegretto Objective WA device works in a way that can be summarized as below: laser 532Nd：YAG projects a parellal 0.3mm-diameter light cluster on the cornea. The laser travels through the pupil with diameter circa 6-7mm into the eye by a grid consisting of 13×13（168）points to project the image onto the cornea. Therefore, digital cameras with aperture（1mm）can capture abnormal images. By means of computer applications provided by the device, we can analyze such images so as to identify the WA[12]. Before taking measures, however, mydriasis condition must be reached because otherwise such image cannot be projected. Pupil size may significantly influence the measuring result of WA. Quoted by other documents, because of the precise construction of the human eye and its strong adjusting capacity; a larger portion of WA can be eliminated under small pupil condition whereas when pupil is large, the effect of WA can be exaggerated by 10-20 times[13], under such circumstances (large pupil), spherical WA may increase significantly. Therefore, only under large pupil condition can all the factors be observed and recorded[14]. During the data collecting process, degree of mydriasis on a particular cataract eye may differ. To those that are difficult to reach the pupil diameter of 6mm or higher, more mydriatic eye drop should be used (15min/dose x 2~3 doses). In case mydriasis still cannot be achieved, the test result on this eye should not count.

WA can be expressed by Zernike multinomial or RMS (root mean square), calculated by wavelength (λ) with measuring unit as µm. (Z_4^0) as the forth coefficient of Zernike and RMS4 (4th root mean square of aberration) indicate the size of aberration. RMSh indicates the overall high-order RMS of the aberration. These three parameters, i.e. (Z_4^0), RMS4 and RMSh, are the major measures in our research. It is observed that (Z_4^0) differs significantly among senior patients who are over 70 years-old (Graph 3-6). Other research papers proved that the irregularity of the corneal surface and broken tear-film are causing factors of a higher-order aberration. To avoid this, we use corneal topology device to look into the surface of the eyeball before conducing objective aberration check. In addition, other factors may also contribute to the final testing result, such as the accuracy and adjusting capacity of WA device, cone cell, and the chosen direction on testing aberration etc[15-17]. During our research, therefore, we use the said criterions to limit our collection only on those reliable and representative data for further analysis.

3.2 Age effect on WA
Age is an important factor causing the aberrations of the human eye, especially spherical aberration. Many researches have proved that along with aging, increase of aberration mostly happens on the vitreous instead of the cornea. Aberration also changes from negative to positive which cannot be offset by the aberration of cornea and ultimately result in an overall aberration increase. Our research analyzes and confirms the correlation between the age factor of 72 patients with their aberration data. Due to limited devices and resources, we did not collect data of spherical aberration on the cornea as from theoretical point of view, aging does not effect corneal aberration in a material manner.

3.3 Effect of aspherical IOL to postoperative WA
Comparing differences of aspherical IOLs (TecnisZ9001) and spherical IOLs (CeeOn Edge911 and Sensar AR40e) taken at one-month, three-months or six-months after surgery, we can see material difference in parameters such as Z_4^0 and RMS4. TecnisZ9001 IOL working mechanism is based on empirical studies done on a comprehensive sampling of corneal and eyeball spherical aberrations of Caucasian patients. TecnisZ9001 is the improved version of conventional IOL so as to offset positive corneal aberration. Our research compares various groups of objective WAs collected before surgery which not only justifies the conclusion that aspherical IOL does reduce postoperative WA but also prevents both false negative and false positive from happening. In our research, we used CeeOn Edge911 IOL as the benchmark and filtered off other technical factors which may effect our testing results (detail please refer to Table2). In doing so, we can further prove the validity of the statement that aspherical IOL does reduce postoperative WA. We also compared SensarAR40e IOL implanted on 32 eyes from 16 patients. SensarAR40e is a typical IOL made from acrylic ester material, which provides the basis for further study on the effects of IOLs of different materials to WA. In addition, only in Group Tecnis Z9001 we saw a significant objective/subjective WA (Table5) after surgery. WAs observed in Group CeeOn Edge911 and Group Sensar AR40e, however, are no material different pre- or post- surgery. This result also proved that compared with spherical IOLs, aspherical IOL has a better effect in reducing the wavefront aberration after surgery.

From a medical perspective, to take full advantage of aspherical IOLs, it would be the trend of its future development for different individual, which closely intertwines with the WA driven cutting (technology?) conducted in corneal refractive surgery. In addition, the physical structure of aspherical IOL can serve as a platform upon which next generation IOLs will be developed. The Tecnis-Array IOL, developed by AMO Com., ltd, that are currently accepted and used by the community, is such an example.

3.4 Effect of aspherical intraocular lens on postoperative visual function
The questionnaire we handed out were designed based a standard VF-14. Modification has been made with

Chinese social condition well considered. Its scoring and scaling system are identical to that of VF-14 which enjoys a high creditability. We believe it is a comprehensive research which well represents the actual visual function of patients in China and therefore presents market value in the future.

Visual function is influenced by many factors. Putting aside the effect from a patient's vision (no material difference was recorded on BCVA taken one month, 3-month and 6-month pre- and post-surgery in Group Tecnis and Group 911, no material difference neither in Group Tecnis and Group Sensar), it is safe to say that apsherical IOL does provide patients with a better vision. As for the study on correlation between WA and visual function, however, we did not receive the expected result and therefore, further study is needed.

3.5 Discussion on our research objects and our methodology

In ideal and hypothetical conditions, study case should be chosen in a complete random manner with a "double-bliend" principle applies throughout the research; only patients with both eyes cataract should be chosen and each of which should be implanted via different IOL. Due to our resource and the same-IOL-on-both-eyes-on-a-single-patient principle, however, we cannot reach the ideal condition and we therefore applied the t-test on two groups of individual samplings. Based on the statistical difference, our clinical study is also able to prove the difference between spherical and aspherical IOLs on their respective reducing power on the WA and improving power of the vision.

3.6 Explanation on the contrast sensitivity result

Illustrated by Graph 7 and Graph 8, compared with the other two groups, we see a high frequency in IOL Group TecnisZ9001. X-axis represents spacial frequency whereas y-axis represents the sensitivity level compared with FACT testing table. Due to limited resources, rigorous restricting on the light condition was not observed but we did adopt a few measurements in our research; including but not limited to 1) tests should be conducted in the same room; 2) with door/windows shut; 3) apply daylight lamp; 3) no logarithmic transformation should be made on the testing results. Because of such conditions, we cannot judge if material difference is out there between impacts of two types of IOL on after-surgery contrast sensitivity. Supported by other papers, however, it is proven that aspherical IOL plays a greater influnece on contrast sensitivity than that played by spherical IOL[18].

Conclusion

The preliminary clinical study, on wavefront aberration affected by a phacomulsitication cataract extraction & intraocular lens implantation surgery, has shown the effect of age to the wavefront aberration of the human eyes. The senior a patient grows into, a greater wavefront aberration is seen in his/her eye.

We are in favor of aspherical IOL, over spherical IOL, in terms of reducing WA; improving contract sensitivity and achieving a better after-surgery visual function.

Bibliography

1. Bailey IL. Visual acuity. In: Benjamin WJ, ed, Borish's Clinical Refraction. Philadelphia, PA, WB Saunders, 1998; 179–202

2. Liang J, Williams DR, Miller DT. Supernormal vision and high- resolution retinal imaging through adaptive optics. J Opt Soc Am A 1997; 2884–2892

3. Alonso J, Espallargues M, Andersen TF, et al. International applicability of the VF-14; an index of visual function in patiens with cataract. Ophthalmology 1997;104:799-807

4. Cassard SD, Patrick DL, Damiano AM, et al. Reproducibility and responsiveness of the VF-14; an index of functional impairment in patients with cataracts. Arch Ophthalmol 1995;133:1508-1513

5. Robert WM, Gary SR. Visual function assessment questionnaires. Surv Ophthalmol 2001;45:531-548

6. He JC, Burns SA, Marcos S. Monochromatic aberrations in the accommodated human eye. J Vision Res,2000;40(1):41-48

7. Burton G, Haig ND. Effects of the Seidel aberrations on visual target discrimination. J Opt Soc AMA,1984;1(4):373-385

8. Liang J, Williams DR. Aberrations and retinal image quality of the normal human eye. J Opt Soc Am A 1997,14(11):2873-2883

9. He JC, Marcos S, Webb RH, et al. Measurement of the wavefront aberration the eye by a fast psychophysical procedure. J Opt Soc Am A Opt Image Sci Vis,1998;15(9):2449-2456

10. Zhu L, Bartsch DU, Freeman WR, et al.Modeling human eye aberrations and their compensation for high-resolution retinal imaging. J Optom Vis Sci,1998;75(11):827-839

11. Applegate RA , Thibos LN , HilmantelG. Optics of aberroscopy and super vision. J Cataract Refract Surg,2001;27:1093-1107

12. Mrochen M, Kaemmerer M, Mierdel P, Krinke HE, Seiler T. Principles of Tscherning aberrometry. J Refract Surg,2000,16:S570-S571

13. Charman WN. Pupil dilation and wavefront aberration. J Refract Surg 2004;20(1):87-88

14. Martinez CE, et al. Efect of pupil dilation on corneal optical aberrations after photorefractive keratectomy. J Arch Ophthalmol,1999;127:1-7

15. Marcos S, Burns SA. On the symmetry between eyes of wavefront aberration and cone directionality. Vision Res, 2000,40:2437-2447

16. Klein SA , Garcia DD. Line of sight and alternative representations of aberrations of the eye. J Refract Surg,2000,16:630-635

17. Schwiegerling J . Theoretical limits to visual performance. Surv Ophthalmol ,2000 ,45 :1392146

18. Mark P, Howard FI, Richard S.H. Improved functional vision with a modified prolate intraocular lens. J Cataract Refract Surg,2004; 30:986-992